The ABCs
Of L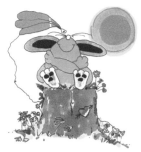ving Yourself
With Diabetes

Inspired living with diabetes

Written & Illustrated
by Riva Greenberg

SPI Management LLC
Brooklyn, New York

SPI Management, LLC
Brooklyn, New York 11215

ISBN 13: 978-0-615-17094-7

Second edition 2009

A portion of the proceeds from this book will be donated
to organizations making life better for those with diabetes.

Text and Illustrations by Riva Greenberg
Editing by Claire Gerus
Design by Bill Greaves

Printed in the United States of America

This book is available at special quantity discounts to use as
premiums and sales promotions. For more information, please
go to: www.diabetesstories.com/abcbook.html

For my father

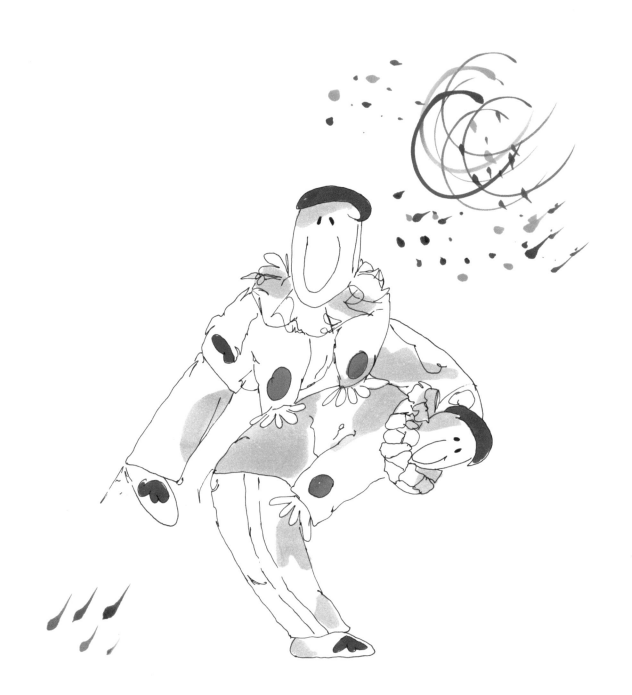

Contents

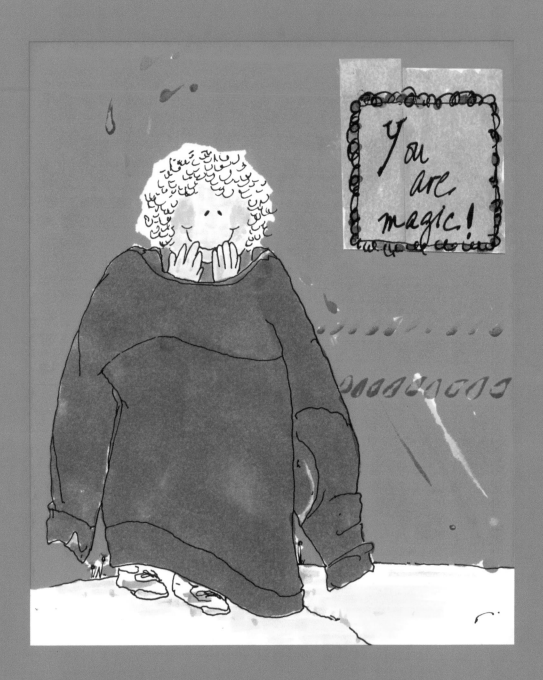

Foreword

The emotional side of diabetes is often ignored or neglected and yet is such a critical part of living with the disease day in and day out. It is easy to get overwhelmed, tired, defeated, frustrated and down about diabetes.

In my work as a clinical psychologist at the Behavioral Diabetes Institute (BDI) we address the emotional and behavioral side of living with diabetes. Through workshops, classes, and discussion groups we offer people a forum within which to share their personal struggles and victories, and discuss and work through difficult emotional issues. Connecting with others who truly understand what it is like to have these thoughts and feelings can cause remarkable transformations. Just knowing that you are not alone with what you are going through, and believing that there is hope in what you are struggling with, can create new ideas, possibilities and motivation.

Sometimes healing needs a change in the way you look at things. It may be looking at your next high blood sugar number and just seeing it as information to inform your next decision, rather than as a judgment of yourself. Or, reminding yourself that it's impossible to "do diabetes" perfectly, and so aim to do your best.

At the BDI we have learned that for many people changing their thoughts and behavior regarding diabetes is a long journey, but as Riva says you can appreciate the steps you take. In the end, living with diabetes means taking responsibility and taking charge. I've seen when people do that, particularly with the emotional issues of living with diabetes, their management improves, which means their day improves and their life improves.

The author and illustrator of this book, Riva Greenberg, inspires others to not just live with diabetes, but to thrive with diabetes. With gentleness and wit she challenges her readers to acknowledge and address difficult emotions in an effort to see that we are worth the hard work of loving ourselves.

—**Susan Guzman, Ph.D.**
   Senior Psychologist
   Behavioral Diabetes Institute
   www.behavioraldiabetes.org

Sometimes the hardest things in life
turn out to be blessings in disguise.

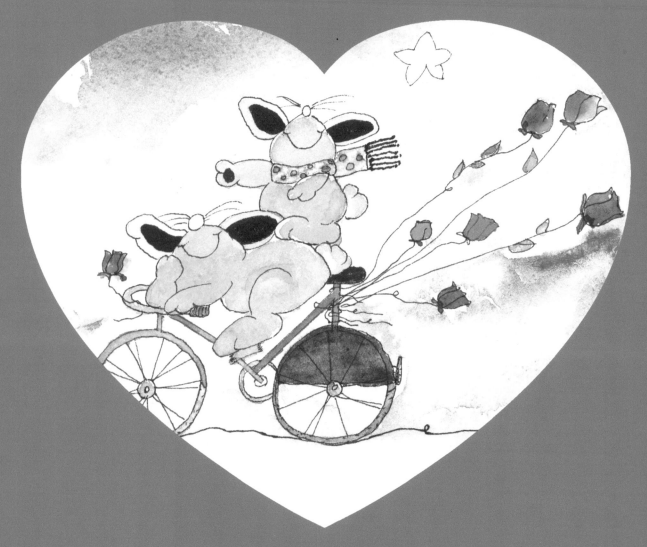

Diabetes can be one of them.

To My Fellow Travelers

At 18, I developed type 1 diabetes. Looking back, it was an odd time. I was not quite an adult, no longer a child. I have now lived with diabetes for more than 37 years, in the beginning not so well, over the years better and better, and now perhaps brilliantly – or fairly close, aware that this chronic condition requires both my medical and emotional attention.

Like so many, I have been through the typical stages: denial, anger, bargaining, depression and acceptance. On some days I go back 'round again. I've enjoyed additional stages like outright disgust, "You don't understand!" and a perfectionist's frustration. However, as I learned more I reached out more, and shifted my focus from hefting the burden of diabetes to seeking ways to ensure my best health. As a result, my A1cs, my attitude, and my responsibility all improved.

Getting married for the first time at 48 was also a driving force to do my best. With added motivation and support, I got behind the wheel of my health and haven't looked back – except to make sure my husband isn't covered in my dust.

I believe all of us with diabetes, and our loved ones, can benefit from the emotional nurturing, spiritual principles, understanding and support you'll find here. It is my hope that this little book will put a tiny "I love me" patch on the hearts of all who read it.

Personally, I view diabetes as a blessing, for I am quite certain without it I would not stick to my daily walking program (particularly on cold, windy days). Nor would I have learned to like vegetables so much, or mastered waving bye-bye to my beloved muffins and scones. Diabetes has also given me my work, wonderful friends who share membership in this club, and the opportunity to contribute to the world and those who live with this disease.

I hope in your journey with diabetes you will arrive at that place, if you haven't already, where diabetes is a "comma" in your life, as in…"I love my life, and I have diabetes." Someone once said this to me and I don't expect to ever forget it.

Learn everything you can, put the pedal to the metal – with your personal mettle on each pedal – and make life as full, rich and exuberant as you deserve. And should some dark clouds pass overhead, give a shout or have a cry, reread a few pages here, and then get on with it.

—Riva Greenberg

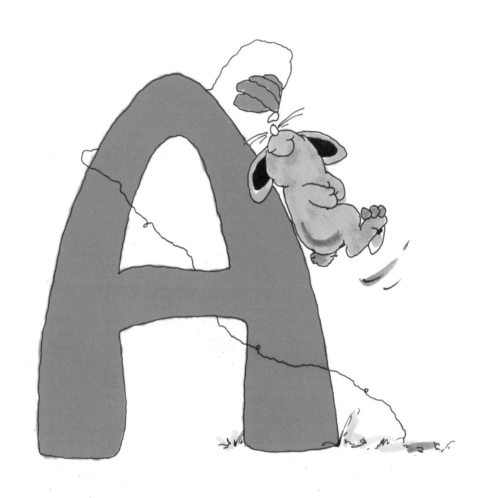

A is for Appreciating All the
Special Things You Are and Have

Life Is a Joyful Blessing

Living with diabetes is something you learn to do each and every day. On some days, you hardly know it's there. On others, you can hardly forget. But appreciation is what fills our lives with love, joy and deep contentment, even when you have diabetes. Appreciation opens your heart to see and experience the goodness in life, filling you with gratitude for what you have. Imagine, diabetes can actually open your "appreciation spout!"

How? First, diabetes can motivate you to make healthier food choices and improve your fitness. Second, you can take pride in how bravely and powerfully you are managing diabetes. And third, when you lose something it's an opportunity to appreciate all the more what you *do* have.

Having diabetes may at times make you feel you've lost some spontaneity, freedom or ease in life. Maybe you're worried about the future or feel there are "rules" you have to live by and things you can't do.

That's not true. You can do and have anything when you make choices that support your best health. Actually, choosing anything less is a disservice to yourself.

If you do feel you've lost something with diabetes, ask yourself if you've gained something too. There is always something gained when you see life through the eyes of appreciation.

Here's an act of appreciation you can perform right now. Think about the people closest to you. Why not write each of them a note, telling them how much they mean to you? When you send love out into the world, it comes back multiplied.

Diabetes can be a gift in your hands if you use it to see how many blessings you truly have: loving family and friends, a dear pet, a comfortable home, the use of your body and mind, meaningful work, a favorite hobby, all your simple pleasures and exuberant passions, and just the marvel of being you.

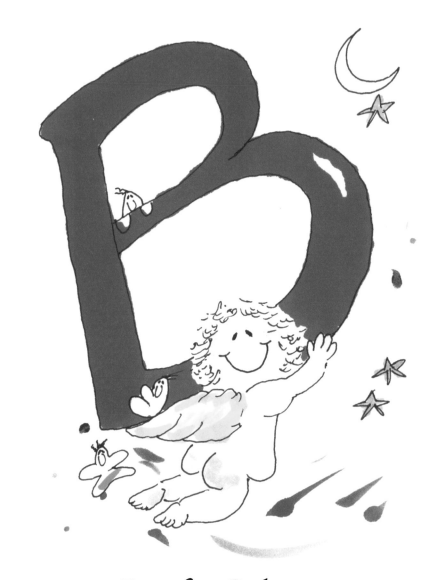

B is for Believing
You Are Stronger than Diabetes

Believe in Your Power

Life will test you; in fact, it probably already has. When life tests you, it's an opportunity to find your inner strength, to renew your resolve, firm up your commitment, clarify what's truly important to you and create new ways to achieve your goals.

A challenge isn't there to stop you, but to help you commit your passion, creativity and spirit to getting where you want to go. Believe that you are stronger than diabetes and you will be!

Why? Because believing will inspire you to take actions that support that belief – actions that will help you best manage your diabetes. Believe in anything and you'll begin to make it so. Believe in yourself and you're creating your own "luck" – you can build a life that's full, rewarding, healthy and happy, regardless of diabetes.

Diabetes may test you, but it will also bring out your true power. Your strength will emerge when you decide to take charge of your own life.

So many people have overcome great obstacles. Thousands of people have performed great athletic feats with physical disabilities. Inventors have defied skeptics and transformed and enriched how we live. Ordinary citizens have stood against oppression and shone a light where only darkness prevailed. Millions have risen from misfortune to become forces for positive change in their communities.

Heroes are not born; they are simply people motivated to do something bigger and better than it was done before.

Having diabetes can be your opportunity to reach for something higher. It can reveal to you just how strong and capable you are. Open your heart to your own possibilities. Focus your attention inside yourself and hear your own wisdom say, "I am powerful, I am capable, I control my diabetes."

Your power to be stronger than diabetes is within you.

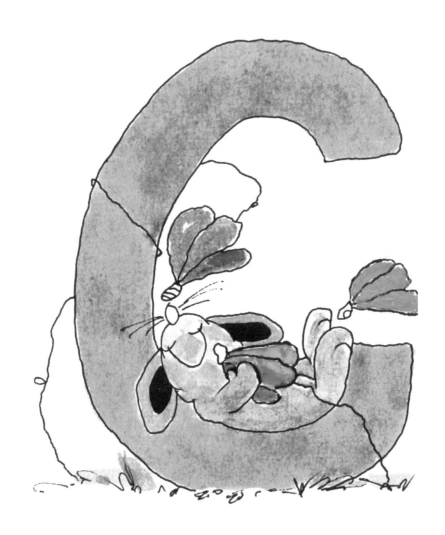

C is for Choosing
a "Can-Do" Attitude

Who "Can-Do?" You Can!

A "Can-Do" attitude is one of the best ways to ensure maximum health. A "Can-Do" attitude energizes and inspires you, and helps put you in charge of your diabetes. You're better able to get through frustrating times, and can make the tough choices when confronted with a brownie à la mode or strawberries à la diet whipped cream. A "Can-Do" attitude *can do* this. Really!

A "Can-Do" attitude is a choice. Sometimes, without realizing it, we choose to take a "victim" attitude about our diabetes, and it stops us from taking good care of ourselves. It's natural to feel down or frustrated at times, so when that happens accept your feelings. It's part of being human. Then, pick yourself up and move on again with "Can-Do-ness."

Decide that you will do what it takes to be as healthy as possible. If you have type 2 diabetes, you can with a little hard work, control it so well you'll hardly know it's there. If you have type 1 and test your blood sugar more often, you'll take fewer rides on that roller-coaster of high/low blood sugars. Now isn't that worth some "Can-Do-ness?"

Keeping yourself healthy may require changing some habits you've had for a long time. But remember, while bad habits, old beliefs, and feeling sorry for yourself may be where you've been, they need not be where you're going. Yesterday is gone. Tomorrow, on the other hand, is being created by every action you take today.

A "Can-Do" attitude is about confidently choosing the actions that will support your best health. Eat more heart-healthy foods to reduce your risk of heart disease. Start a walking program to lower your chance of foot problems.

And finally, remember that stopping along the way to smell the flowers and appreciate life's simple pleasures keeps "Can-Doers," "Can-Doing."

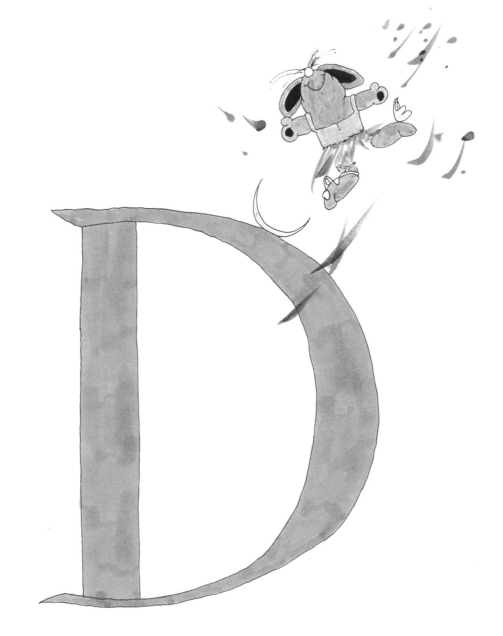

D is for Dancing
Your Unique Dance through Life

You Have Something to Do Here

It is no accident that you are here now. You have something special to contribute to the world through the unique talents and gifts you have been given. Maybe you are meant to do something on the world stage – something that changes people's lives on a grand scale. Maybe you are meant to change the world, person by person, by taking extra care and time for those in your life.

Many people use their diabetes as a stimulus to live more giving lives, understanding better than others that life is precious.

It's easy to get caught up in today's frenetic pace and the "To-Dos" that constantly crowd our lists. Think about turning your list onto the other side. It's blank, isn't it? Ask yourself, while looking at that empty sheet, "How can I contribute to the world? What am I good at? What do I love to do? How can I better the lives of my family members and friends? How can I create a difference in my community?"

Athletes, artists, inventors, philanthropists and others in all walks of life, have become role models by how they live their lives with diabetes. Many use their diabetes as a platform to teach others and show the world that while diabetes may challenge us, it does not stop us or make us any less than anyone else.

How you live your life every day can serve as an example to others. Perhaps what you're here to do is simply be the best person you can be. Maybe you can be even stronger in your character, gentler in your actions and kinder to those you encounter.

When you dance your unique dance through life with diabetes, you inspire everyone, not just those who have diabetes. That's the gift you give to others just by being you!

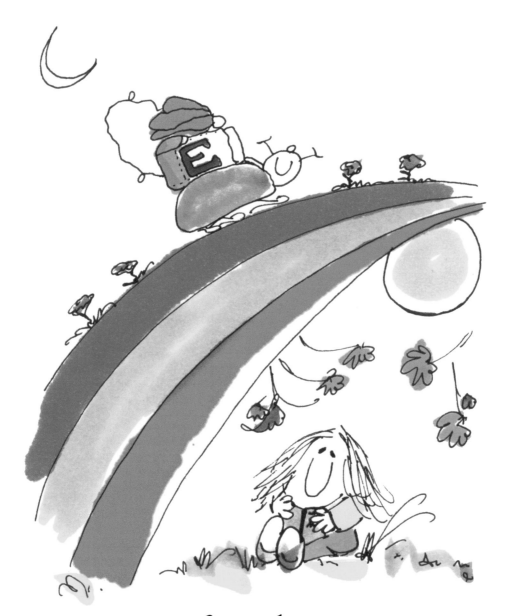

E is for Education.
It's a Major Step to Success

Knowledge Is Powerful Medicine

Learning how to take care of your diabetes is one of the best investments you can make toward living healthfully. Many people think taking care of their diabetes is up to their doctor or diabetes educator. But it's not. They're not with you during the day to remind you to perform your diabetes tasks – to test your blood sugar or choose broccoli over French fries. Diabetes needs to be managed every day by the person who has it – you.

Learning as much as you can about diabetes and the importance of controlling your blood sugar is one secret to living a full and healthy life. There may be much to learn, but you can do it. Think back to a time when you learned something that you knew very little about. Perhaps it involved a project at work, a volunteer job or studying a new subject. In the beginning, you may have been a little intimidated by how much you didn't know.

But in time, you learned. And then, you relaxed. You gained new insight, new understanding and new skills. What felt like an uncomfortable stretch, over time became easy and familiar. This is how taking care of your diabetes will become when you educate yourself about it.

Think about this: Going through life without knowing how to control your diabetes is like boarding a bus whose driver is wearing a blindfold – you just know you're going to run into trouble. On the other hand, there's a lot you can do to stay healthy when you know how.

Here are a few starters: Ask your doctor questions and write down the answers. Subscribe to a diabetes magazine. Check out the internet or join a support group.

Get "diabetes smart" for knowledge really is power. More than that, it's powerful medicine.

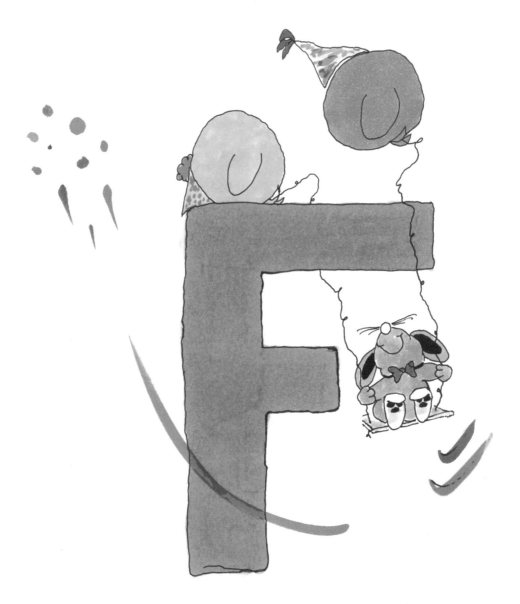

F is for Having Faith in
Yourself, and in a Higher Power

The Power of Faith

Faith is believing that even when the world is not treating you well you will be all right. Faith is a direct channel to your inner strength and wisdom; it is a force that can help you accomplish almost anything.

However, whether you have your faith turned on or not is another matter. You need to have faith, now, that you can meet the challenge of diabetes.

When you have faith, you understand that you do not walk alone. A Higher Power works through you and walks alongside you. Don't let your faith be beaten down by someone you knew who suffered with diabetes. They may have lacked faith and so didn't make the best choices. They may not have had the benefit of all that's available today to help manage diabetes. No matter what, know that there are gifts to be found when you walk this road in faith.

What's important now is to put away your worries and trust yourself. Know that you have an inner well of strength to draw on whenever you may need it. Right now recall a time when you brought your heart and passion to something so fervently, you didn't doubt yourself or that you would succeed. Decide now that you will bring this same spirit to how you manage your diabetes.

How do you do this? By "acting as if." That means you act as if what you want is already so. If you "act as if" you are successful managing your diabetes you will be. You will naturally take the steps that will produce this. Then, even the occasional bump in the road will merely show you how capable you are of overcoming it. Embrace living well with diabetes in your heart and you will see it play out in your life.

If you have faith in the work you do to keep your diabetes in good control, your results will reflect it. If faith can move mountains, it can certainly move you can't it? Let it lift you today to bring back your confidence and vitality.

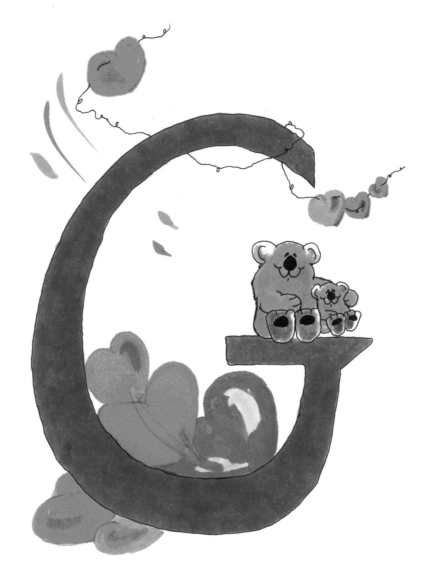

G is for Grabbing onto Hope
for You and Your Little One

You Can Be a Calm Parent

Any parent knows that the worst thing about diabetes is that it strikes children. Type 1 diabetes usually occurs in little ones and changes their lives forever. Children with diabetes must watch what they eat, take daily injections or wear a pump, and always be vigilant to avoid low blood sugar and losing consciousness.

For parents, diabetes can feel like the death of your dream – a child who's happy, healthy and has every opportunity. The theft of childhood, a new family dynamic, finding the right doctors, exhaustion and worry are now fixed aspects of your life.

You may even feel guilty. You may believe that you let your child down by missing the warning signs of diabetes, or think that you caused your child to get sick. Know that this is not your fault; you couldn't have prevented it. Forgive yourself if need be and do your best to care for your child.

You are the source of your child's strength, confidence, guidance and support. Know too that children come through this. Many say they are stronger, more appreciative of life and more compassionate because they have diabetes.

Take action to help yourself restore a sense of normalcy. Talk with your child's teachers and classmates to educate them about diabetes. Dispelling fear goes a long way toward creating a supportive environment for your child. Start a support group where resources, feelings and friendships can be shared. Don't neglect your other children – celebrate special days to honor each one of them.

Then when it's time, give your child the space to make diabetes his or her own. Until then, try to make life for all of you about *more* than diabetes. Remember, children take their cues from you, and every day remarkable things are happening to change the face of diabetes. Let a positive face be the one your child sees when he or she looks up into yours.

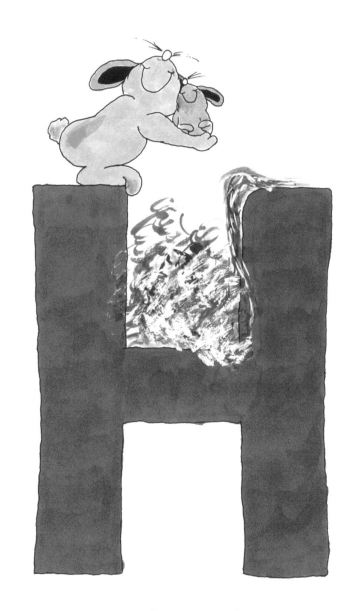

H is for Helping
Others Help You

Create a Team Around You

Many of us go through life feeling we must shoulder our troubles alone. We think it is weak to ask for help. We may even take pride in doing everything for and by ourselves. But that's a very poor way to manage diabetes and it puts you at risk. Diabetes affects many bodily functions, as well as emotions and stress levels. Having a team of health care providers to help you manage your diabetes can be invaluable.

Did you know the word "team" also stands for "together everyone achieves more?" This is so true. Rarely can one person achieve as much as a group. Think of your diabetes specialists as your personal team. Each member of the team is there to assist you in gaining greater control by contributing his or her unique talent.

Team members support, encourage and inspire each other. Don't hesitate to go to one of your team if you're having difficulty. Never forget, too, that you are a member of this team. It is your responsibility to participate in your care and use the team's guidance wisely.

Joining a support group is another great way to extend your team. Members share lots of information, and who better can understand the ups and downs of living with diabetes than those who have it? Friends or family members can also be part of your team.

Don't underestimate the power of a team. Studies show that people with diabetes do better when they work with team mates. Remember, too, having a team is not an act of weakness, but one of taking responsibility.

After all, you earn a badge of courage every day when you live with diabetes. Now, be courageous enough to let those trained to help you do exactly that.

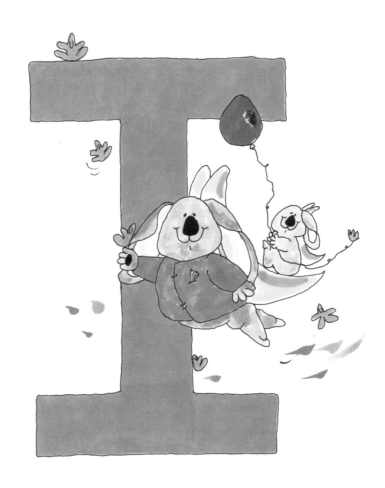

I is for Intention, Invention,
Illumination and Inspiration.
With These You Can Fly High

Let Your Energy Lift You

Often in life even when you don't know how you're going to accomplish something, you discover that just by having a firm *intention*, the "how" to get the job done shows up. You see with new eyes, hidden doors seem to open, and solutions appear out of nowhere. Intention is so powerful that just by intending to better control your diabetes, you will. Why? Because you will naturally take the steps that support this intention.

Invention can also help you with your diabetes management. You can invent yourself anew as someone who manages diabetes well. See yourself in this new role by holding a mental picture of being a diabetes "pro." See yourself performing your tasks effortlessly. Feel how relaxed and confident you are. You can become better at managing your diabetes by returning to these images often, or simply by taking healthier actions. Either way, you'll be on the path to becoming a new you.

Now let's look at the power of *illumination*. You are illuminated, lit from within, when you realize something. For instance, if you know you don't test your blood sugar as often as you should, or that you could be doing better with portion control, allow that truth to burn so brightly that it burns right through all your excuses – and ignites your intention to do better.

Last comes *inspiration*. Inspiration is a sense of excitement and purpose that comes from the center of your being. Inspiration unleashes your confidence, strength and power to get the job done. To connect with your inspiration, think about what gives your life meaning and purpose.

Intention, invention, illumination and inspiration are powerful energy forces, and are an intrinsic part of who you are. If you begin to trust them and invest in them, they can help you accomplish magical results beyond your wildest imagination.

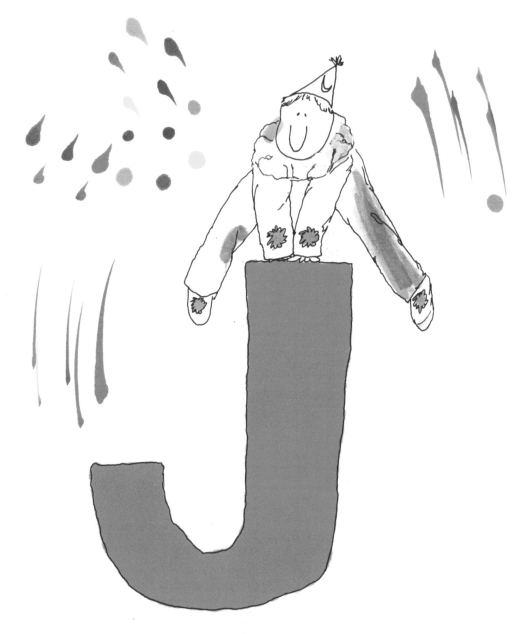

J is for Joy.
It's a Powerful Healer

Laugh Loudly, Fully and Often

You know that when living with diabetes, diet, exercise and medication may be a necessary part of managing your condition. In addition, there are other healing agents that are often overlooked. These won't cause you any inconvenience or discomfort and you can take them any time of day. These healing agents are happiness, laughter and joy. These actually increase the level of "feel-good" hormones in your body, which can help your cells repair and renew themselves.

A big belly laugh, researchers say, releases a hormone that keeps your immune system healthy. So stack up some funny movies for tonight because, amazing as it sounds, just anticipating a good laugh has significant neuroendocrine effects.

Huh? Yes, just anticipating happiness triggers a cascade of beneficial physiological changes. It's like smiling. When you smile, a warmth begins in your heart and spreads through the rest of your body. You immediately feel a sense of happiness, peace and calm.

Norman Cousins, noted author and editor-in-chief of the *Saturday Review*, also became famous for his personal "laugh cure." While suffering with a severe illness, he hired a nurse to read funny stories to him and play Marx Brothers movies for him. His laughter relieved his pain and he made a complete recovery.

At the time, Cousins received a good deal of skepticism. But in 1989, the *Journal of the American Medical Association*, acknowledged that laughter therapy could help improve the quality of life for patients with chronic illness.

Here's something else you should know. Joy, happiness and laughter are not something you *find* in life, but something you *bring* to life. So stop to see the magic of a snowflake, and laugh 'til the tears run down your cheeks. Look for the funny, sunny side of life. You'll be giving yourself a powerful booster shot of health.

Note: You can take joy without a prescription – so start today!

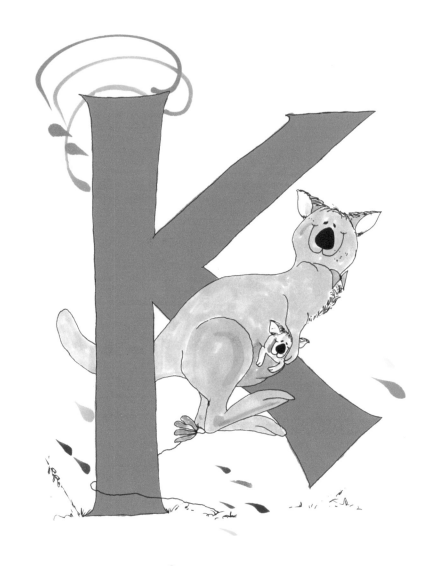

K is for Knowing
You Are Capable of Change

Shift Your Attitude

No matter how long you've had diabetes, if you aren't taking good care of yourself you can do better right now. Whether you've spent years ignoring your doctor's advice or even avoiding your doctor, today you can decide you will be the master of your diabetes, not the other way around. The first thing to do is to decide what you truly want. Chances are, that's to live as healthy a life as possible as long as possible.

The second thing that will benefit you is to shift your thinking. Rather than seeing your diabetes care as something you *have* to do, see it as something you *choose* to do.

In other words, if you're saying to yourself, "I *have* to test my blood sugar, I *have* to lose weight, I *have* to exercise," you feel as if you're being forced by someone else to do these things. However, if you say to yourself, "I *choose* to test my blood sugar," you feel in control.

Then, recognize the benefit of actually doing the task. For instance, "By testing my blood sugar, I can keep it in target range and reduce my risk of complications." Focusing on the benefit will help remind you why the task is important.

The truth is, everything we do in life is a choice. We say, "I have to" about many things, but there is really nothing we "have to" do. You may think you "have to" go to work, but you don't. You may lose your job if you don't go, but you don't "have to" go. Rather, every morning you "choose to" go for your own personal reasons.

Changing your mindset from "have to" to "choose to" will empower you in your diabetes care, and in your life. With all there is to be gained, isn't it time you hopped to it?

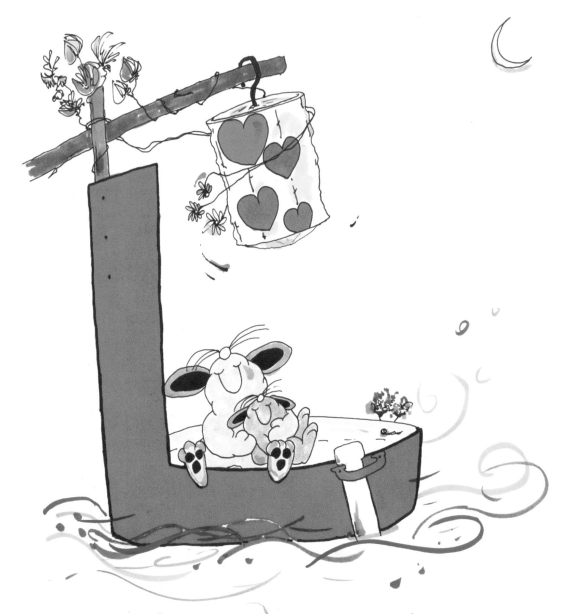

L is for Love. Let It Lighten
Your Load and Light Your Way

Know that You're Not Alone

Your diabetes doesn't just affect you, it also affects those who love you. They know you have something extra you carry on your shoulders each day. They may see you struggle at times and not know how to help you. But they're with you, anyway.

Your loved ones need to have a role in your diabetes care; they need to know how they can help you. Set aside a time to sit down and talk with them. Together, you will find ways that they can be of practical and emotional support.

Pick a comfortable setting and a restful time to talk honestly with your loved ones. Open your heart about what living with diabetes is like. Also, let your loved ones open their hearts, for you are all in this together. Then help them understand how you feel, what's easy, what's hard, how much effort diabetes takes, what you wish you were better at, and any guilt you carry or fears you may have.

Next, explore what they can do that would be helpful for you. Perhaps they can prepare healthier meals if they do the cooking. Maybe they can take a walk with you after dinner so you get regular exercise, or see that your diabetes supplies are always stocked. Maybe they can just listen when you feel down. Let them know a little extra kindness and being sensitive to your feelings goes a very long way.

Then expand your support circle. When friends invite you for dinner and ask what you can eat, be honest with them. They only want to make things easier for you. Tell a colleague at work what to do if you should experience low blood sugar. Their intervention could be vitally important some day.

A medical team will light your way as far as guiding your care. Having a personal support team goes a long way towards lightening your load.

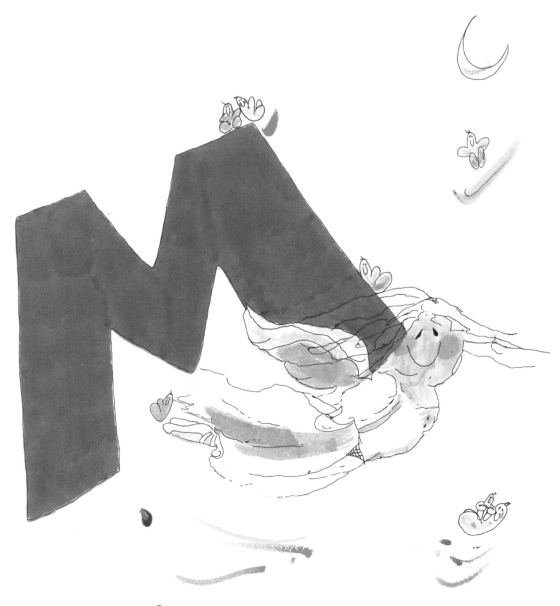

M is for Magic. You Create It
by Believing in Yourself

Create Your Own Magic

Here's the secret ingredient to making magic happen: believe in yourself. You are an incredible, talented, capable, loving person, but do you know it? Do you treat yourself with the same regard, kindness and compassion you reserve for a friend? You deserve no less! How you feel about yourself influences how well you will take care of yourself.

When you believe in yourself, you live life expecting the best. When you exude confidence, the world responds by rewarding you with a very special magic. This does not mean you will always succeed, but failing does not make you a failure. There are lessons to be learned when you fail, and learning from your mistakes brings a special kind of magic too.

If life has convinced you that you are not worth believing in, your vision has been clouded. When you wake in the morning before you open your eyes, take two minutes and look within. See on the screen of your mind your strengths, your talents and your gifts. Picture yourself at your best. Do the same in the evening before you drift off to sleep. Magic will be set into motion even as you sleep.

If you have spent much of your life saying "yes" to everyone around you, leaving you little time and energy for yourself, practice saying "no." You can't truly take care of anyone else when your own energy is depleted. And if your past has not reflected your greatness or your ability to manage your diabetes, remind yourself with love, that today is a new day; today you will take a new step.

The world only reflects back to you how you see yourself. Therefore, see yourself as someone who can manage diabetes well. This is how you can create true magic in your life.

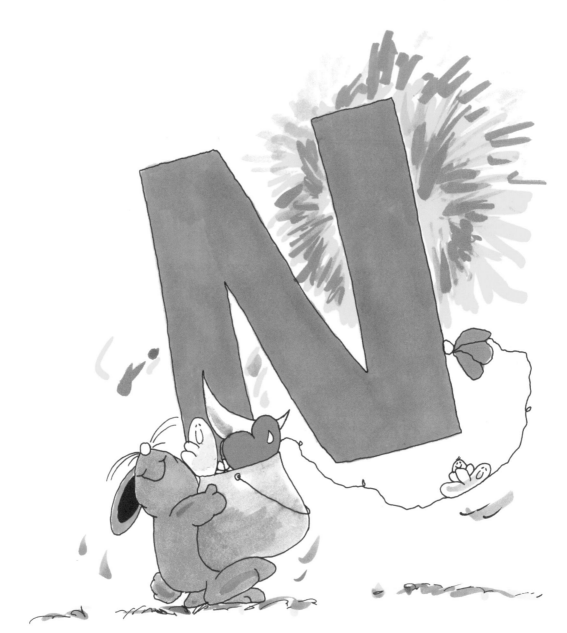

N is for Nurturing Yourself
Whenever You Need It

Give Your Spirits a Lift

Diabetes may get you down at times from the work it takes and the fears of an uncertain future. When it all feels like too much, do something you love to do. Relax in a scented bubble bath, go to the movies, gaze up at the stars, spend a weekend with a gripping mystery novel, or an evening with a friend who fills your heart while you pour yours out.

Since life with diabetes never gives you a day off, you may occasionally have to give yourself one. Just as people take vacations from their jobs, you may need a vacation from your diabetes. That could mean having dessert once a week, or skipping a blood sugar test now and then. Just be sure to choose something that gives you a break, but doesn't put you in peril.

It shouldn't be a long vacation; just a brief rest to recharge your batteries. Like any satisfying vacation, plan ahead and know where you can safely stretch yourself. Nurturing yourself and taking planned mini-vacations can help let off some steam. This may help you manage your diabetes care better over the years.

If, however, you seem to have lost your zest for life, feel down, sleep too much and avoid your friends, you may be experiencing depression. One-third of people with diabetes at some time experience depression. Physical activity and being with others can help shake off the blues – if that's all it is. But if your mood's unshakeable, you may need professional help. If you are depressed, both your blood sugars and your life will be hard to manage.

Week to week, if you do things you enjoy, take brief vacations, treat yourself kindly, and avoid dwelling on things that make you sad or angry, you'll find the spring is back in your step before you ever lose it.

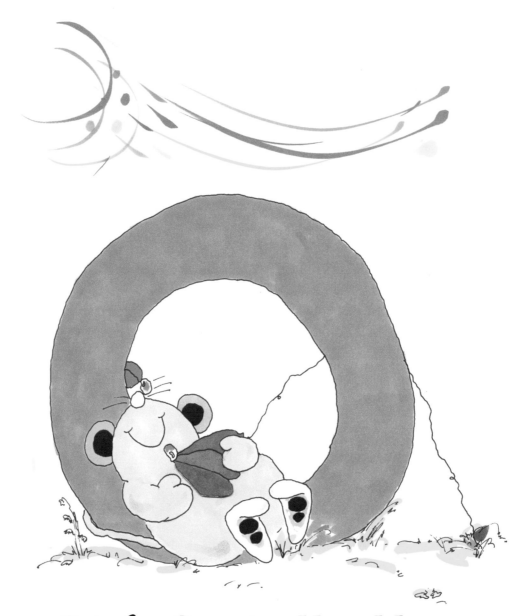

O is for Opening Your Heart
and Letting Yourself in

Give Up the Guilts

People with diabetes often live with a good deal of guilt. You may think you actually caused your diabetes by eating too many sweets. (That's not how one gets diabetes.) Type 2 diabetes tends to be genetic, and type 1 is an autoimmune disorder.

You may feel guilty if you do not expertly manage the many tasks diabetes requires. But even experts say this can be difficult. Since guilt is not productive, appreciate that diabetes is not an exact science; no matter how hard you work at controlling it at times it will foil you. Keep your spirits up and experiment with different practices.

Guilt steals your energy; it robs you of feeling happy and contented, being truly present for your loved ones, and above all it interferes with your taking care of your diabetes. Let the guilt go. Know that you will have good days and bad, including days you'll overeat, are too tired to exercise, will shout at your spouse and receive blood sugar numbers you don't like. Just make sure those days don't turn into weeks and months.

Diabetes is not who you are; it is something you are learning to live with. It does not make you damaged, or broken, or unlovable or any less a person. It's not easy being on patrol 24/7, 365 days a year.

Love yourself more fully because you are doing your best, whatever that happens to be right now. Forgive yourself when things go awry. And accept yourself as the uniquely amazing person you are with all your gifts, and yes, faults, too.

Living with diabetes takes extra energy, awareness and commitment to your health. So open your heart and let yourself in all the way. When you do, you'll discover you have an infinite supply of love and resourcefulness to support you every day, even living with diabetes.

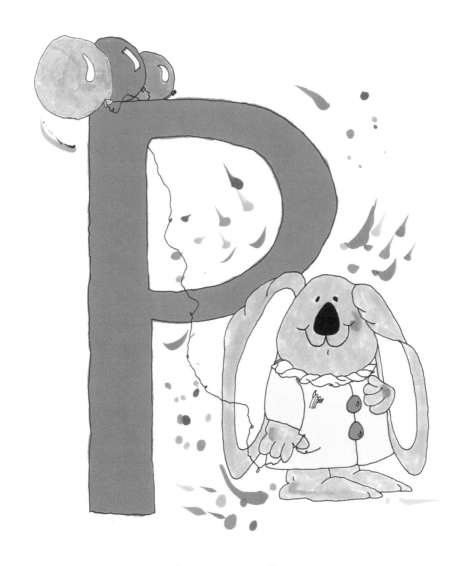

P is for Perfection
and Knowing It's Not the Goal

Good Can Be Great

So many of us strive for perfection in our work, in our family lives, and in our diabetes care. But the truth is, perfection is unattainable. You can't eat perfectly every day, at times an event will prevent you from exercising, and your blood sugars won't be perfect every single time. No matter what you do, striving for perfection will often leave you feeling like a failure.

There are so many tasks involved in taking care of diabetes that it's just not possible to do them all perfectly. Then there are the times your body will unwittingly sabotage you.

Human beings are simply imperfect. There is always something more we can learn and something more we can do to improve. Trying to be perfect extracts a very high price. It can cost you your peace of mind and cause you to give up entirely because you can't meet your own high expectations. Further, it limits what you are willing to try since you are wedded to the result being perfect.

Perfection is not the goal to aim for. Rather, try to do well most of the time. What's important is doing the best you can each day and being honest with yourself – you know when you're doing less than you should.

Remember, too, that balance is important. Life shouldn't be all work. In fact, enjoying yourself, playing, laughing and giving yourself occasional "diabetes breaks" are all good medicine.

Doing well with diabetes, not perfectly, should be your goal. You may have to lower your bar, but you will feel more satisfied with yourself and everything you do. Then, embrace your own perfection simply by being the unique creature that you are. Perfection is unattainable, but being pretty darn good, now that's something to shoot for!

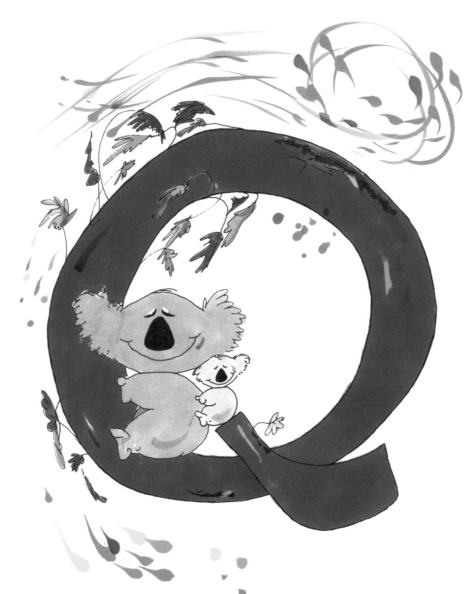

Q is for that Quiet Place that
Offers Shelter Against a Storm

Peace and Tranquility Await You

Some days are harder than others when you live with diabetes. You may already be living with some complications, and then there are so many things you need to do. It's like there's a ticker-tape in your head constantly calculating meal times, pill times, up times and down times. There's the 100th diet you've tried and fallen off of – again. Sometimes diabetes is just a pain to live with, not unlike a houseguest who never leaves.

At these times, you need a place to retreat to where you can take a "time out." There is such a place; a kind of paradise where peace and tranquility await you. You won't have to pack a bag or rush to the airport because this peaceful place exists within you.

Some people experience this place in meditation or yoga, lying on a beach or losing themselves in a daydream. You can also experience this calm and tranquility by stopping whatever you are doing, taking a few deep, slow breaths, and getting more oxygen into your lungs. Peace really is that close at hand. When everything outside you feels overwhelming take shelter within.

Here is your personal, private sanctuary. Here lies your true self; your spirit, gifts, talents, creativity, love and untapped potential. Here you are whole, complete and perfect. Moreover, here you can let go of all your worries and fears. You can recharge, revitalize, and return to the world rested, with greater clarity, awareness, energy and resolve.

When diabetes seems to fight you, get you down, seem impossible to control, be unfair, ruin your day, your peace, and every attempt you make to manage it, go inside. Be still and connect with your inner strength. It is your anchor in the storm of life. It will shield, restore and recharge you each and every time.

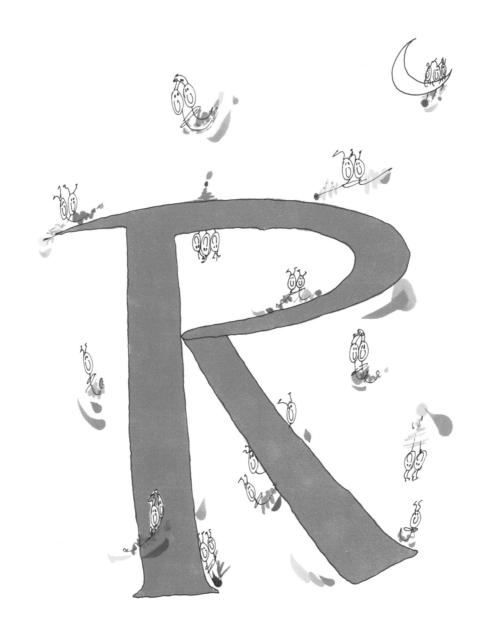

R is for Rejoicing
that Diabetes Is Manageable

You Are Truly Fortunate

You can live a long and healthy life with diabetes if you take care of it. Imagine for a moment that your doctor just told you that you had an illness for which nothing could be done, and you only had six months to live. Many people are not as lucky as you.

Many diabetes practitioners consider diabetes not an illness, but a condition you can learn to live well with. Diabetes requires work; that's true. But that work can keep you healthier in the long run. Taking care of your diabetes may actually safeguard you from developing something worse.

Creating a treatment plan with your doctor that's right for you, and keeping a positive outlook, go a long way toward being healthy with diabetes. And while diabetes calls for extra effort and attention, don't put your life on hold. Stay busy making your dreams happen. You'll find the pleasure and energy your dreams give you make your daily diabetes tasks easier to do.

Think too, where can you combine your diabetes management with some fun? For instance, can you call a friend to be your walking buddy or dance partner? Look for ways to enhance your enjoyment of life while improving your health. Then sing, cheer and be grateful!

Many diabetes professionals feel that if you keep your blood sugar in good control you can live a long and healthy life. Now isn't that cause for celebration?

If you haven't made a commitment to your health yet, make it now. And every day turn negative thoughts around by giving thanks that you have a condition that's manageable. By regarding diabetes more positively you'll see that joy, delight, pleasure and happiness are buzzing all around you.

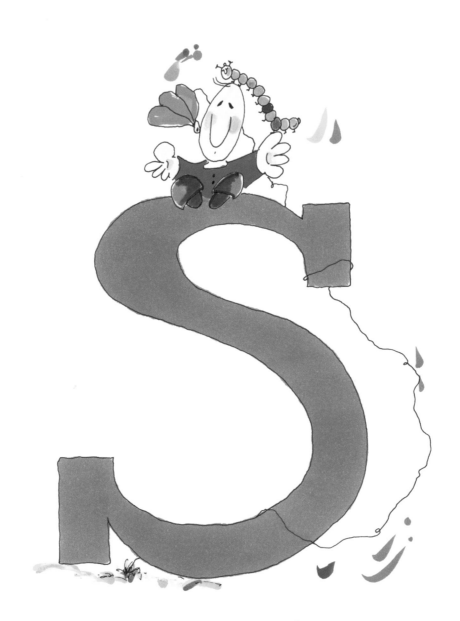

S is for Small Changes
that Create Big Results

Take One Step at a Time

Most people find it difficult to make changes. It's easy to get stuck in habitual ways of doing things and often hard to get unstuck. Perhaps you think a change has to be an entire overhaul, or should be done with lightning speed. Not true. The best way to make any change is to break it down into small steps and take one step at a time. Once you take a small step and enjoy your success, you'll feel confident to take another.

Sometimes changes are hard to make because you fear the unknown. Most people take comfort in familiarity, even when what they are doing isn't working very well. You may be surprised to know that while change seems to take a lot of energy, doing the same thing again and again without success may deplete your energy even more.

Ask yourself, "What one small change can I make today to take better care of my diabetes?" For instance, if you'd like to incorporate more exercise into your day, you can begin with a short walk, perhaps in the morning or after dinner. While you do this, adopt an attitude of "practice" with your change, then *slowly* increase your walks in length or speed.

Any change you make is better begun small. Tackling something too big can set you up for failure, whereas small changes made incrementally larger set the stage for success.

Here's another tip: while you're mastering a change reward yourself, not for your results, but for having the courage to take new action. This keeps you moving in the right direction and it sends a signal to yourself that you are, indeed, capable of change.

So rev up your commitment, perseverance and determination, and always keep your goal in front of you. Before long, your small changes will pay off in big benefits!

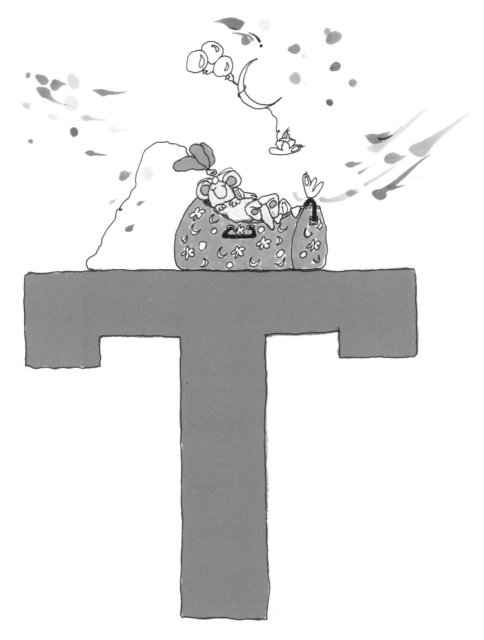

T is for Thanking Your Lucky Stars that You Have Diabetes – Now

There's New Research Every Day

In the last five to ten years, there have been more advances in treating diabetes than in the past fifty! In fact, it's remarkable how much has become available today to help you manage your diabetes.

Fortunately, and unfortunately, the increase of diabetes around the world has led to a wealth of new medicines, devices, approaches and research that offer greater health. There is also a greater focus on helping people manage the emotions that may arise having diabetes.

Living with a chronic illness can, at times, make you feel depressed, angry, frustrated, fearful or fatigued. These emotions are important to manage so that they don't interfere with performing your diabetes tasks. One quick way to lift your spirits is to give thanks for how much easier diabetes is to manage today than just a few decades ago.

Imagine, 40 years ago those living with diabetes had to more precisely time their medicine to their meals and eat snacks even when they didn't want them. They had to boil syringes and needles in a pot on top of the stove. And one never knew one's blood sugar because home meters didn't exist.

Compare that scenario with today's lifestyle. Now you can test your blood sugar at any moment. There are also treatment strategies like carbohydrate counting, and food labels actually list carbohydrates. There are disposable syringes and new medical procedures for old problems like vision loss. There are pumps that calculate food's impact on blood sugar and continuous glucose sensors. There are people who have become insulin-free through islet cell transplantation. And every day, stem cell research brings greater understanding and hope for a cure.

If you feel sad or overwhelmed at times having diabetes, acknowledge your feelings. Then remember that today you can live a full, rich and long life with diabetes. For that, you can thank your lucky stars!

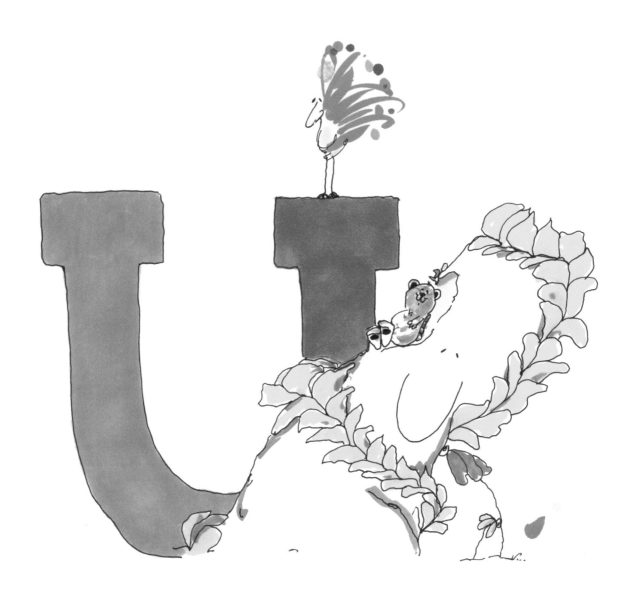

U is for Understanding
that Life Has a Perfect Rhythm

On the Road to Acceptance

Like many people, when you first discovered you had diabetes you may have experienced a profound sense of loss. You may have felt that spontaneity had left your life. This is not uncommon, nor is experiencing the 5 stages of grief – denial, anger, bargaining, depression and acceptance – as you learn to integrate diabetes into your life. What's important is traveling through the stages and arriving at the final one, where diabetes is not your enemy, but a part of you and how you live.

Denial is a common reaction to diabetes. At times denial can protect us, but not when it comes to diabetes. If you can't admit you have diabetes, you will not put the appropriate effort into managing it.

Anger often follows denial. You feel, *I don't deserve diabetes! It's not fair!!!* Anger creates enormous stress on your body, mind and spirit.

Next may come bargaining. *"Oh, please, if you take away my diabetes, I'll never complain again..."* But bargaining will not make diabetes go away.

Depression is very common with diabetes. You feel, *Why bother? It's too much. What's the point?* Like denial, if you are suffering from depression, it is almost impossible to take care of your diabetes.

Acceptance is the last stage of grieving and the first in turning a new page. You feel you can take care of your diabetes and live a happy life, regardless of its presence.

Just as life has cycles, so too will living with diabetes. There'll be stormy periods and then the sun will come out again. You may move through a stage and then fall back in unexpectedly.

Don't be surprised when this happens. Just make sure that you give grief the heave-ho as soon as you can. There comes a natural time to let go of grieving so you can move on and more successfully manage your diabetes.

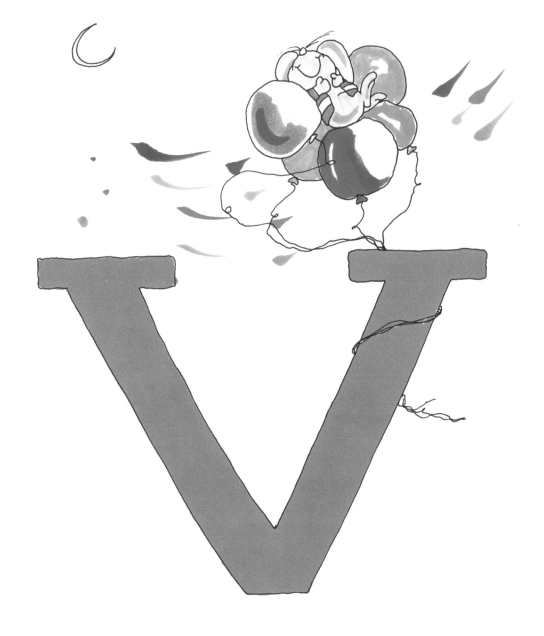

V is for Victory.
It's Yours with a Plan

Create a Road Map to Success

Having a personal action plan – one you create yourself that inspires you – is one of the most effective ways to help you manage diabetes. Your plan should contain a big goal you want to accomplish. For instance, it could be to lower your A1c (average blood glucose level) or practice healthier habits. Often people are afraid to set goals because they fear they won't achieve them. But not having goals is a sure-fire way to achieve very little.

Choose a goal that excites you, because accomplishing it will require both your time and effort. Write your goal down. This helps make it clear and motivating. Then create a vision of having achieved your goal and feel the happiness you expect it will bring you.

Next, list the steps you will take toward achieving your goal. These steps create a road map to follow. Just as you'd check a map to see what streets to take when driving to a new place, your action steps are the map to your goal.

Sometimes when you're working toward your goal, you may do less than your best or feel like giving up. At these times, remember why you chose this goal. Its meaning and importance to you are likely to re-inspire you.

As you work with your plan and take new steps, celebrate your progress. You might put a gold star next to each step you accomplish. When you've accumulated three stars reward yourself. A bouquet of your favorite flowers, a day at the museum or a long, leisurely lunch with a friend are lovely ways to celebrate success.

With a carefully conceived plan, *victory* – enjoying your best health – can be yours. Don't wait, start creating your plan today. After all, there's no time like the present to give yourself this very special gift.

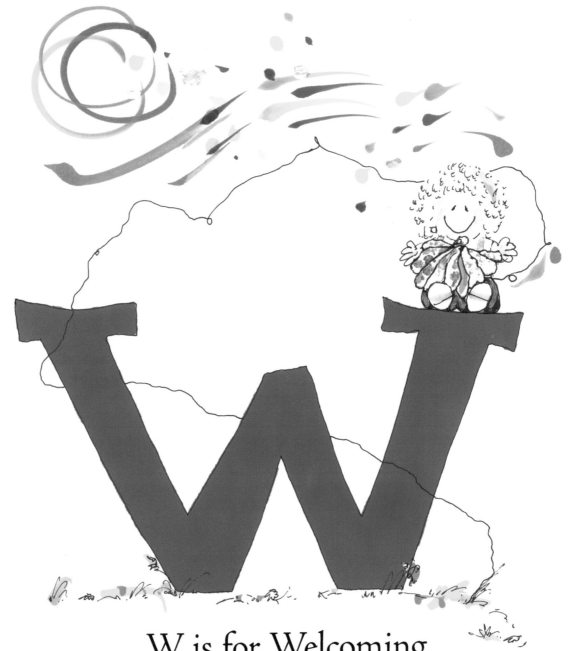

W is for Welcoming
Your Absolute Best Health

Make All Your Actions Count

Every day, the actions you take and don't take contribute to your health. Turning your actions into healthy habits is one way to better manage your diabetes. Like all habits, healthy habits can save you time and effort and free you to enjoy your life outside of diabetes. Never forget, that's an important part of living well with diabetes.

Creating an environment that supports your efforts is extremely helpful too. For example, can you make your home more diabetes-friendly? Clearing the cupboards of junk food and filling them instead with fruits and vegetables is a great start. How about keeping a calendar especially for doctor visits and filling prescriptions?

You can put structures in place that support you outside your home as well. Regard your health care providers as partners helping you achieve your best health, and work with them to design a treatment plan that you can manage. Invite a friend to exercise regularly with you. It's great motivation and a lot more fun. Remember, above all else, the actions you take every day create the fabric of your life and your health.

There's yet another place to find support when managing your diabetes feels like too much work. That's within yourself. Think about why you want to be healthy. What gets you excited in life? Who are the people you love? The answers to these questions will remind you why it's worth staying the course.

Your actions, attitude, determination and willingness to do your best create your health each and every day. No matter how many times you've failed, it does not mean you will fail again. Develop an unshakeable desire to succeed and chances are you will.

When you make your actions count, you open your arms to your best health – today, tomorrow and for all the years to come.

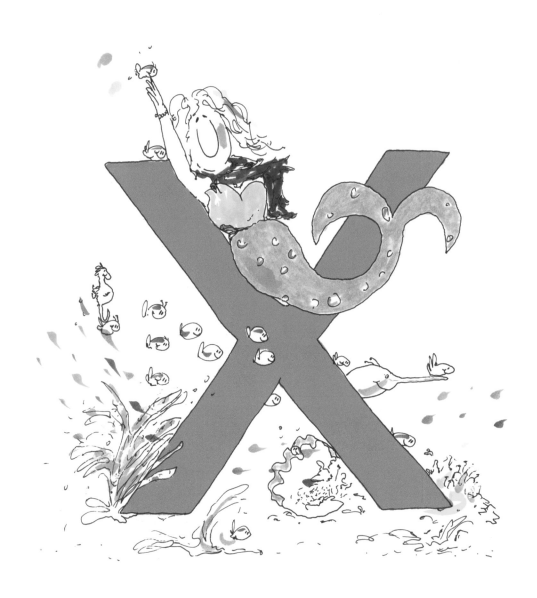

X is for the Xtraordinary
Creature You Are

Anything Is Possible

Gary Hall, winner of ten Olympic medals, learned how to manage his diabetes so he could continue swimming competitively. Amazingly, he improved his technique and swims even faster with diabetes. As a spokesperson for diabetes research, Gary often says that with the right tools and information anything is possible.

Last year, Will Cross became the first person with diabetes to reach the South Pole. Will is a world-class mountain climber and a popular motivational speaker. He's devoted his life to demonstrating how goal-setting, preparation and determination can overcome seemingly insurmountable obstacles – even with diabetes.

The legendary blues guitarist and winner of nine Grammys, B.B. King, spent much of his career traveling across the country by bus, performing with type 2 diabetes that he's had for over 25 years. Now in his 80s, King continues to inspire fellow musicians and diabetics with his dedication to both his work and his diabetes care.

Golfer Kelli Kuehne, 23, diagnosed with type 1 diabetes at age 10, is a two-time U.S. Women's Amateur champion. Golf World magazine says Kelli is "the best thing to happen to women's golf." Kuehne says diabetes has taught her much about life, discipline, patience, perseverance, adversity and tenacity.

Did you know tennis legend Arthur Ashe, NBA superstar, Adam Morrison, athletes Sugar Ray and Jackie Robinson, inventor Thomas Edison, performers Halle Berry, Mary Tyler Moore, Nick Jonas, Patti LaBelle, Delta Burke and Neil Young, Miss America's Nicole Johnson, entrepreneurs Howard Hughes and Ray Kroc, political leaders Mikhail Gorbachev, Menachem Begin and Mike Huckabee are among the many, many people who live, or have lived, with diabetes?

Today, people with diabetes are winning marathons and triathlons, dancing on the professional stage, jet-setting, running international businesses and making their dreams come true.

What's your dream?

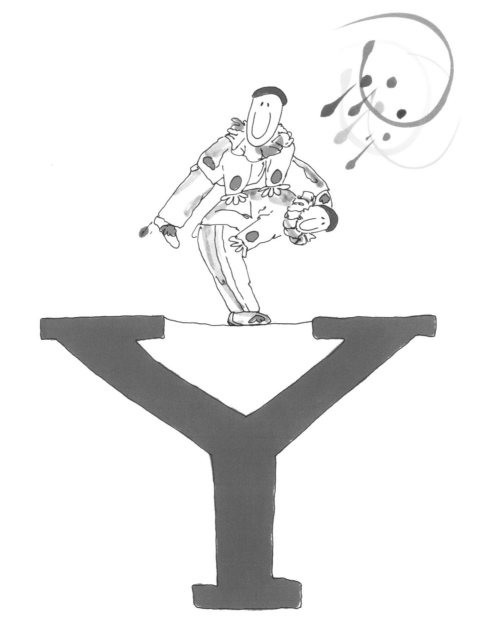

Y is for Saying, "Yes,
I Have Diabetes and a Great Life"

What Do You Love?

Diabetes is handled best when you make it a *part* of your life, not the *whole* of it. You are so much more than your diabetes. Think about what makes your life joyful and meaningful, and find ways to continue doing those things. Life can be as exciting, rich, fun and filled with possibilities as it was before you got diabetes.

What do you love? Are you doing it? Regularly? If not, why not? Doing what you love makes life fulfilling. What you put your attention on tends to grow. Put your attention on being sad, frustrated or angry, and life will become a series of unhappy events. But put your attention on what you love and happiness will come flying back riding full-speed atop the wind's tail.

If you take care of your diabetes there's no reason why you can't enjoy everything you used to. You can also create new pleasures and adventures. Perhaps you've dreamed of going on a wildlife safari, learning how to fly a plane or soaring across a high wire. Maybe turning your passion for gardening into a flourishing new business makes your heart go pitter-pat, or learning to paint or tutor children.

Discover what you love, and hold close the special moments in life you cherish: sitting down to Thanksgiving dinner, playing with your grandchildren, watching the first bloom of spring flowers, feeling your loved one's arm around your shoulder and hearing the words, "I love you."

When you feel down on your luck, you can be high on life again in no time. Accept the here and now and intend your future to be as big, bright and beautiful as you ever dreamed it – or more so. Begin right now by remembering what you love to do, and then doing it.

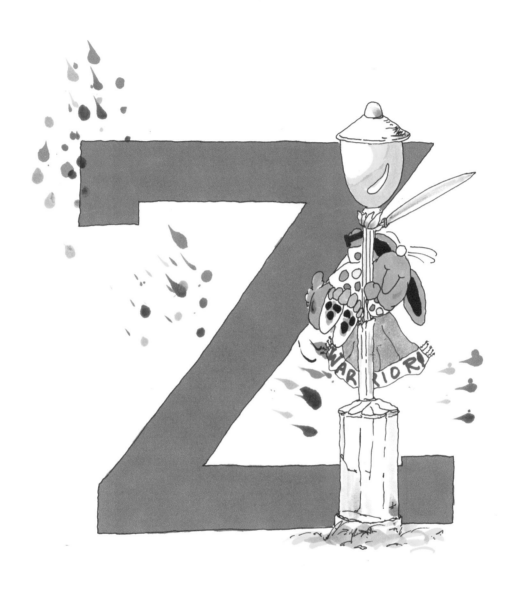

Z is for Zeal.
Every Superhero Has It

Be a Warrior, Not a Worrier

Life with diabetes has its own inherent ups and downs. Some days you feel like you're making mistakes all over the place. Other days you feel like a superhero – managing everything effortlessly. Yet, like a superhero out of costume, no one even seems to notice the battle you fight. In truth, every day you walk a line between being a warrior and a worrier in how you manage your diabetes.

It's so easy to be a worrier. It happens when you let your imagination get the best of you, and let your fears about diabetes get the worst of you. It happens when you're frustrated by the extra work diabetes takes, on top of the work your life takes. When you notice your worrier dominate your thinking, schedule activities that make you happy. This will shift your focus and bring balance back into your life.

Then call out your warrior. Warriors come forth when they sense you are excited about your life, and when they feel your courage and commitment to living well with diabetes. Truth be told, your warrior or superhero may not brandish a sword, fly through the night sky, wear a cape or have webby fingers and toes. However, *Warrior Power* is remarkable, and is activated when you put more faith in being a warrior than in being a worrier.

Wherever you are on your journey of living with diabetes, you have reason to be proud. Diabetes is a special challenge you have been given and you are working at rising to it. Even on tough days, remember that there's a superhero within you.

So get zealous about your care and welcome every day as the gift that it is. It will pay you back with a life filled with even more joy, magic, passion, accomplishment and good health than you could ever imagine!

About the Author, Riva Greenberg

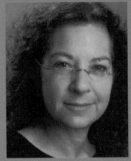

At 50, after living with diabetes for 32 years, Riva decided to combine her knowledge of diabetes care with her writing and artistic abilities. After two decades as a copywriter and change communication consultant, today she is educating and inspiring others to live an exceptional life—not *despite* having diabetes, but *because* of it—through her art, books, blog, research and lectures across the country.

Riva contributes to *DiabetesHealth* magazine and is often featured on their web site. She is also the published author of *The ABC of Loving Yourself.* This is Riva's second book, and the first of several forthcoming books on "living well with diabetes."

In 2009 Riva's book, *50 Diabetes Myths That Can Ruin Your Life: And the 50 Diabetes Truths That Can Save It* will be published. In 2008 Riva won 1st place in the "Inspired by Diabetes" Creative Expression Competition sponsored by Eli Lilly and the International Diabetes Federation.

Riva is an "A1c Champion" with Patient Mentor Institute and a support team member of Divabetics. She also serves on the editorial committee of the Juvenile Diabetes Research Foundation International in New York City and is an Advisory Board Member to Mount Sinai's Diabetes Center and Methodist Hospital's Diabetes Education and Research Center in New York City.

Married to a Dutchman, travel is high on her list of pleasures and diabetes she says, "just comes along for the ride."

To learn more about Riva's work and read her blog, visit her web site at: www.diabetesstories.com. A portion of the proceeds from the sale of this book were donated in 2008 to Diabetes Research Institute, and will be donated again this year to an organization making life better for those living with diabetes.

Acknowledgments

I wish to express my gratitude to my friends and fellow type 1s and type 2s who reviewed this book and made it better – Cindy Stutzer, Phyllis Kornbluth, Carol Weber, Ruth Charne, Pat Molnar Michel Legrou and Yumiko Hara, my fellow A1c Champions teaching others how to live better with diabetes; and my gal pals at Patient Mentor Institute for their support.

Special thanks go to Heather Nichol, RN, MScN, CDE at British Columbia's Children's Hospital and Betsy Rustad, BS, RN, CDE, who lent their professional expertise to this project, my editor, agent and new friend in the desert, Claire Gerus, and my book designer, Bill Greaves.

I thank my unofficial mentors whose teachings have guided me through my life, among them Wayne Dyer, Deepak Chopra and Eckhart Tolle. Some of the concepts in this book come from their shared wisdom. I thank, too, Dr. William Polonsky and Dr. Susan Guzman of the Behavioral Diabetes Institute, whose work has enriched my journey living with diabetes.

Lastly, I thank my husband, who continues to give me unwavering support and encourages me every day in this endeavor.

—Riva Greenberg

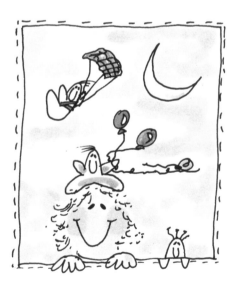

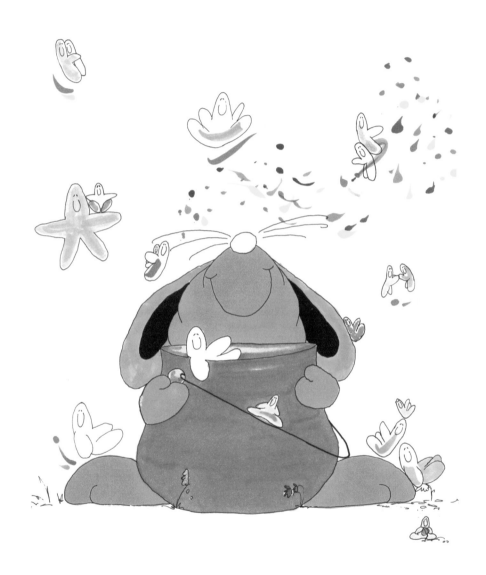

CPSIA information can be obtained
at www.ICGtesting.com
Printed in the USA
BVHW021959170122
626367BV00004B/2